25 DAYS WEIGHT LOSS CHALLENGE

How TO LOSS WEIGHT IN 25 DAYS WITH DAILY SIMPLY HEALTHY HABITS

D. Stanly Kothem

Content

INTRODUCTION

You deserve to feel strong and confident in your body — period! There's nothing wrong with wanting to lose some weight or tone up a little. But, let us be clear, losing weight is not synonymous with restrictive diets, excessive exercise, and negative self-talk. In fact, if you want to lose weight in a healthy, sustainable way, you'll want to do the exact opposite! Forget the tedious calorie counting, long hours at the gym, and self-criticism. And please, don't fall victim to the fad diets and social media-endorsed weight loss products. Instead, show your body some love. Fill your diet with nourishing foods, and exercise because it feels good — physically and mentally — and show yourself some grace and gratitude. Research shows restrictive diets aren't sustainable long-term, anyway! So if you want to lose weight (and keep it off), a slow, steady, and healthy approach is the answer.

How do you get started with a healthy and sustainable weight loss approach? Great question.! This challenge is full of easy-to-implement tips that will help you feel incredible in your body, both inside and out. No restrictions, no gimmicks, no quick fixes! This challenge is simply here to kickstart your weight loss journey by providing you with healthy habits that you can take into everyday life. Because the little things — like sleep, hydration, and stress reduction — all make a big difference when it comes to weight loss! So, really, this challenge isn't just about weight loss. It's about a commitment to a healthier you! Ready to get started? Day one, here we come

Day #1: GET CLEAR ON YOUR WEIGHT LOSS GOALS

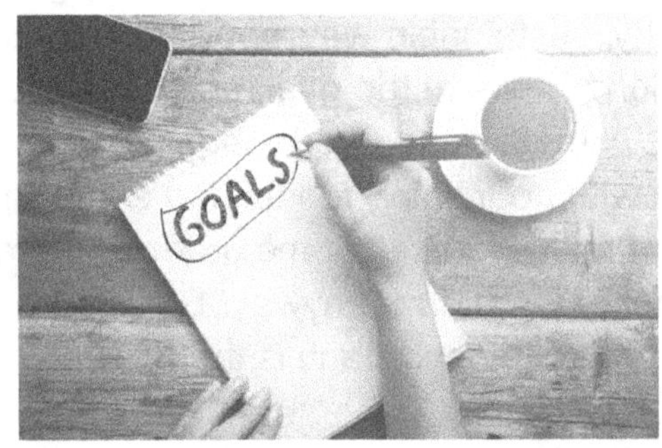

Step one: set your weight loss goals! Before you embark on this weight loss journey, you need to know your 'why.' Take some time with this. Why do you want to lose weight? Do you want to feel stronger or more confident in your body? Do you want to reduce your risk for chronic illness or improve upon the current symptoms you're experiencing? These goals should be about you — not your friend, neighbor, or that social media influencer you idolize. This is your journey!

You'll notice we didn't tell you to set the amount of weight you want to lose. Why? Because again, this is a journey. For some, having a target number may help. If that's you, feel free to add this in! For others, it's easy to get fixated on hitting your goal weight and lose sight of all your other progress in the process. Remember: your weight can fluctuate based on the time of day, how hydrated you are, what you ate, and, for women, where you're at in your cycle. So instead, try setting your goals based on your 'why' and see how that feels!

Day #2: DO A PANTRY CLEANOUT

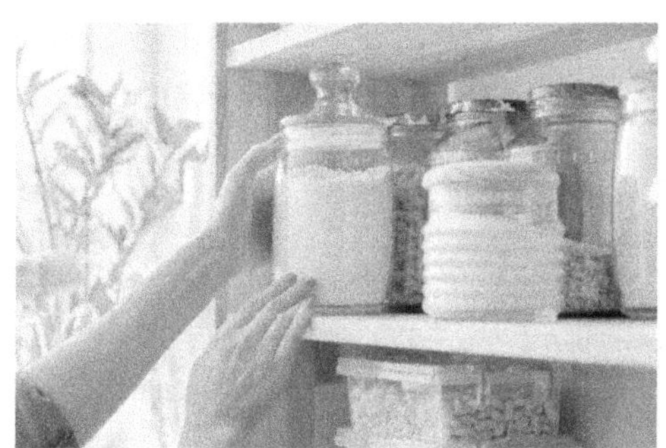

First things first, do a thorough inventory of your pantry, fridge, and kitchen. Toss any expired products, and take note of what foods you have. And make sure to read the ingredient labels! Consider which products contain sneaky sugars, oils, and additives and which products are made with wholesome ingredients. Then, do a quick scan of everything you have — what's the ratio of junk food to healthy food?

While we're not saying you need to toss anything that's unhealthy, try to be mindful about the foods you're keeping. If products are full of ingredients you can't recognize or pronounce, they're probably not going to serve you and your weight loss goals. Toss or donate what you deem appropriate for you and your needs, and make a list of anything that is missing or needs restocking!

Day #3: FILL YOUR FRIDGE

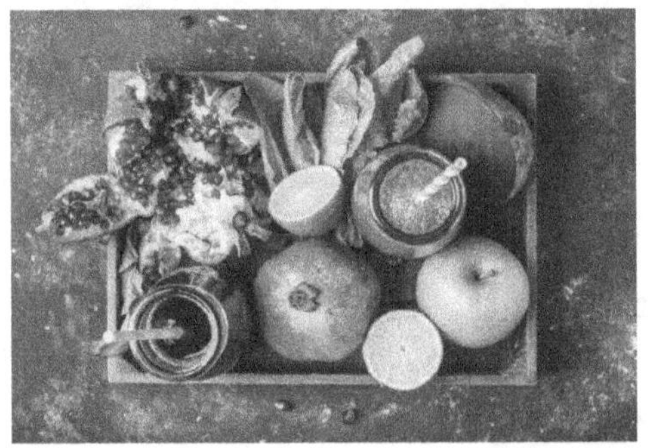

Now that you've cleaned out your pantry, it's time to load up your kitchen with nutrient-dense foods! But before you head to the grocery store, eat a snack or meal! A simple weight loss tip: don't grocery shop hungry! Research shows you'll wind up buying higher-calorie foods based on your cravings and even be more likely to splurge and spend more money than usual.

Instead, fill your fridge with nutrient-dense staples, such as:

Healthy canned goods (chickpeas, beans, wild-caught tuna, and salmon)
Seasonal produce (while considering the Dirty Dozen and Clean 15)
Healthy pasta alternatives (like chickpea and lentil!)
Whole grains and complex carbs (like quinoa and sweet potatoes)
Frozen fruits and veggies (they're cheaper and just as nutritious)

Day #4:START YOUR DAY WITH A GLASS OF WATER

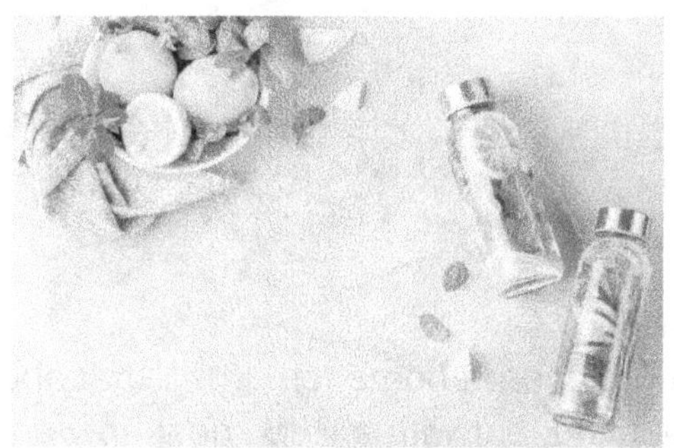

And make it a permanent part of your daily routine! Remember: small, actionable steps make for long-lasting changes. This habit may seem simple, but it sets the tone for your entire day! Plus, drinking a glass of water first thing helps to jumpstart your metabolism and, according to research, even reduces your daily calorie intake.

And if you're a coffee drinker, starting with water can help counteract the dehydrating effects of coffee (since coffee is a diuretic).

You can add lemon, enjoy your morning beverage as a warm herbal tea, or just drink it plain! Include this healthy hack today, but also try to make this a non-negotiable every day

Day #5: COOK DINNER AT HOME

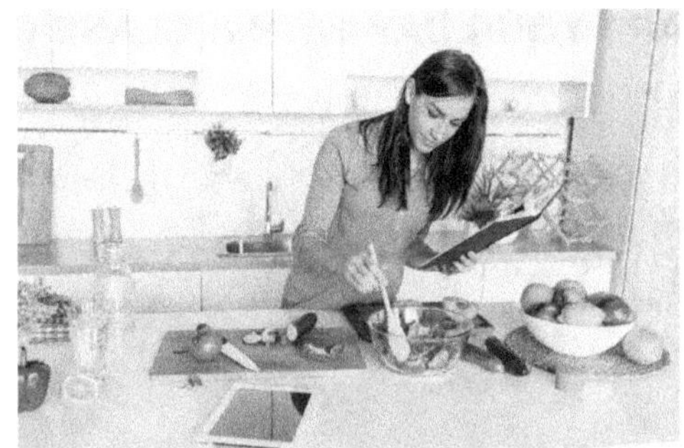

Can you commit to cooking dinner at home tonight? What about for the duration of this challenge? It may sound daunting, but with a little know-how and prep work, it is a lot more manageable than you think! The secret? Calling on techniques like batch cooking, meal prep, and one-pan dinners. Cooking dinner at home allows you to control the ingredients in your food. You can avoid all those sneaky sugars, oils, and sodium while loading up your recipes with nourishing whole-food ingredients.

Here are some of our favorites.

- Dinners Made With One-Pot, Pan, or Baking Sheet:
- One-Pan Herb Crusted Salmon With Sweet Potatoes & Greens
- One-Pot Vegetarian Lentil Curry
- Simple Sheet Pan Tofu Fajitas

10-Ingredient or Less Dinner Recipes

- Broccoli Pesto & Cheese Quesadillas
- Zucchini Parmesan Boats
- Creamy Tuscan White Bean & Artichoke Skillet

Quick & Easy Options: On the Table In 10-Minutes

- Quick & Easy Black Bean Tacos
- Lemon Pepper Shrimp and Roasted Broccoli
- Asian Noodle Salad with Creamy Almond Dressing

Day #6: WALK 5 EXTRA MINUTES PER DAY

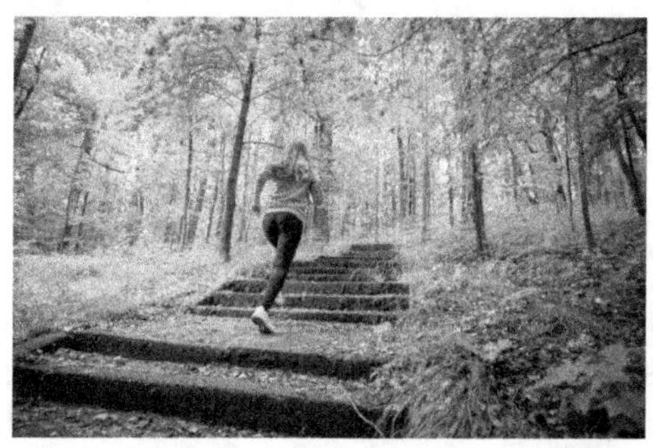

Commit to walking five additional minutes per day — yep, that's it! If you had already planned to walk to the coffee shop, walk an additional five minutes. If you went for a run, add a five-minute cool-down walk to the end of your workout. And if your schedule is jam-packed and a five-minute walk is the only exercise you can squeeze in, that's great too! The idea here is to make these five additional minutes intentional. Again, it may not seem like a lot, but it adds up! Five extra minutes per day (on top of anything you had planned) is 35 extra minutes per week and 140 extra minutes per month. Plus, it guarantees daily movement — even if it's just five minutes.

Start this today, and try to continue this healthy weight loss habit! Once five minutes feels simple for you, add on another five!

Remember: small, actionable goals are the ones that stick

Day #7: MAKE BREAKFAST A PRIORITY

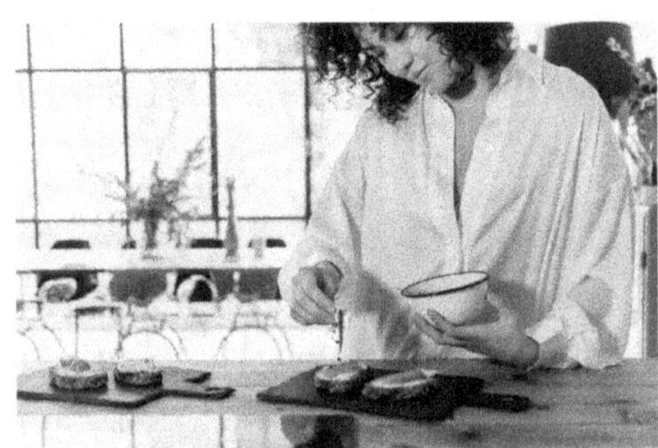

If you're ditching breakfast in hopes of shedding some unwanted pounds, you may want to rethink this decision. There's research to suggest skipping your morning meal increases the risk of weight gain. And I mean, breakfast is the best meal of the day! Oat bowls, eggs, pancakes, smoothies… What could be better?

In all honesty, starting the day with a healthy and wholesome breakfast is one of the best things you can do for your mind and body. A nourishing breakfast helps to curb cravings and increase satiety, it provides you with the energy and nutrients to kickstart your day, and according to research, it leads to overall healthier habits.

Here are some weight loss-friendly ideas, even for the busiest of mornings:

•Make a protein-rich yogurt bowl with Greek or coconut yogurt, fresh or frozen berries, and a drizzle of nut butter.

•Scramble some eggs with a handful of greens, fresh or dried herbs, and any leftover pre-prepped veggies. Serve with avocado and a piece of fruit!

•Heat up a 2-Minute Blueberry Oatmeal Mug Muffin for a protein-packed breakfast that comes together in minutes.

•Toss your favorite fruits, veggies, greens, and superfoods into the blender and whip up a nutrient-dense morning shake

Day #8: MEAL PREP FOR THE WORK WEEK

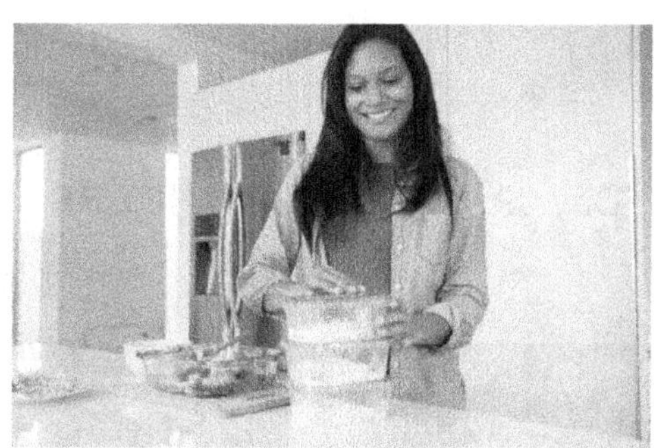

Planning and prepping your meals ahead of time is so important when trying to lose weight — especially during the busy work week. If you have healthy meals prepped and ready to be enjoyed, you'll be less likely to hit the drive-thru on your way to work or Postmate an impulsive takeout order after a long day. Challenge yourself to prep breakfast, lunch, and snack options for the week ahead! Can you continue this through the next 30 days? A little dedicated meal-prep time goes a long way.

Here are some easy-prep FitOn PRO recipes to inspire all your needs:

Easy-Prep Breakfast Options
Make Blueberry Almond Overnight Oats or choose from a variety of flavors
Prep Egg muffins and load them up with your favorite veggies & greens
Blend up some make-ahead smoothie packs and pop them in the blender when you need a quick and effortless healthy option
Make-Ahead Lunch Options
Make this meal-prep-friendly Veggie & Chickpea pasta salad and enjoy it hot or cold!
Whip up a Protein Bistro Box and fill it with your favorite fixings
Prep some quinoa and lentil Vegetarian Lettuce Cups and serve it with a side of avocado and Greek yogurt dressing
Satiating & Energizing Healthy Snacks
Make a homemade trail mix full of nuts, seeds, and superfood add-ins like cacao nibs, goji berries, and unsweetened coconut flakes
Prep some protein-packed Peanut Butter Bliss Balls for an at-the-office snack or an on-the-go pre or post-workout energy boost
Make a simple healthy hummus or guac and pack a serving to enjoy with a side of sliced veggies

Day #9: **SLEEP FOR 8 HOURS**

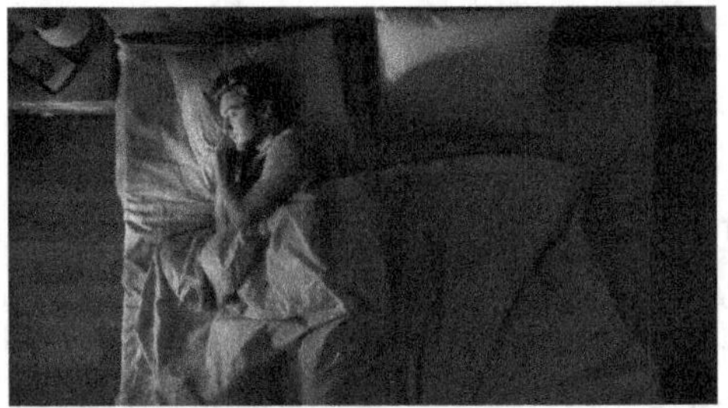

Did you know there's a direct connection between sleep and weight loss? That's right — if you're skimping on sleep, it affects more than just your mood and energy! According to research, 8 hours of sleep (or more) could support your weight loss goals. How so? Increasing your time on the pillow can help reduce the number of calories consumed — an average of 270 calories per night for those who slept 8.5 hours or more!

Sleep deprivation, on the other hand? Not so great. It can trigger hormonal imbalances, such as increased cortisol — a stress hormone associated with weight gain. With sleep loss, you'll also see a reduction in leptin (your satiety hormone) and an increase in ghrelin (your hunger hormone).

The takeaway? Sleep deprivation can sabotage your weight loss success. Try to make this healthy habit a priority — tonight, during the duration of this challenge, + beyond!

Day #10: PLAN YOUR WEEKLY WORKOUT SCHEDULE

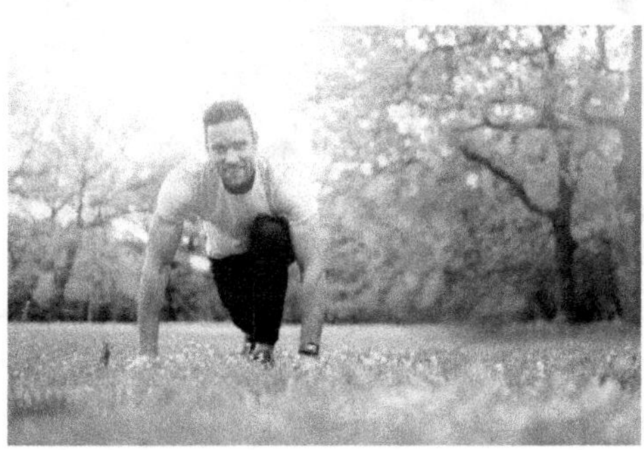

Weight loss aside, regularly moving your body is important. For today's challenge, set aside time to plan your weekly workout schedule. Try to exercise 3-5 times per week, incorporating a mix of strength, cardio, and recovery days. Just as you would a meeting or appointment, schedule your workouts! The more precise you can make it, the better.

Here are some ideas to help keep you accountable:

- Choose a FitOn workout and schedule a reminder in the app
- Join a FitOn Program that's specific to your goals
- Ask a friend to join in on your workout

Planning your workout schedule in advance will help you stay consistent. The benefits? You'll burn more calories, boost your metabolism, and build lean muscle mass!

Day #11: MAKE A HEALTHY FOOD SWAP

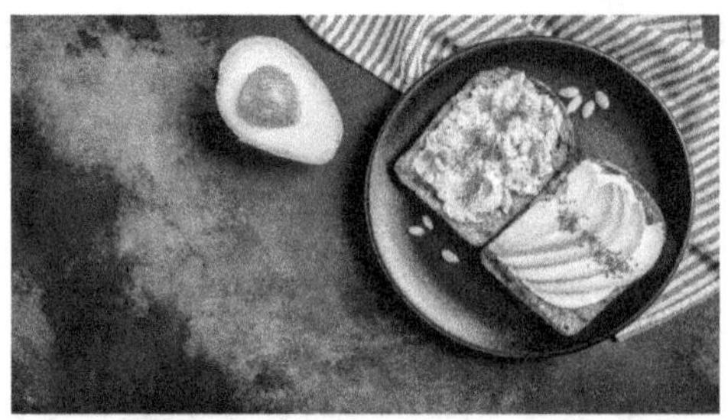

Instead of restricting your diet and eliminating your favorite foods, try calling on healthy food swaps! Your goal today is to tackle one ingredient or food only. Maybe you swap your daily soda for a probiotic-rich seltzer or fruit-infused water. Maybe you make your own healthy coffee creamer instead of the sugar-filled store-bought version you typically enjoy. Maybe you replace your favorite pasta dinner for a healthier twist made with a chickpea pasta alternative.

Rather than trying to change your diet in totality, start with one or two food swaps. Once you feel solid, then add another! Before you know it, you'll have made dozens of healthy swaps that feel manageable. This is the secret to long-lasting changes.

Here are some food swaps that can support your weight loss efforts:

Use mashed avocado in place of mayo, butter, and cream cheese
Spiralize veggies (like zucchini, carrots, and squash) in place of spaghetti and processed pasta
Skip deep-fried french fries for oven-baked parsnip, carrot, sweet potato, or zucchini fries
Blend up a homemade nut or seed-based milk or creamer in place of dairy milk
Swap sugar-filled soda for herbal iced tea, seltzer, cold-pressed juice, or coconut water

Day #12: DO A MINDFUL MEDITATION

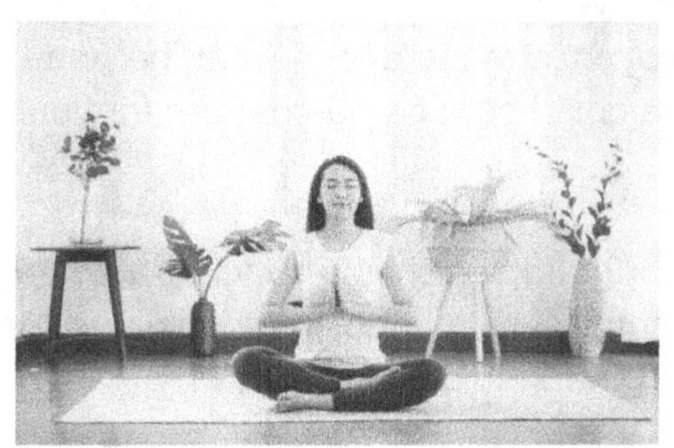

As you may know, meditation is one of the best wellness hacks for stress. While chronic stress is problematic for many reasons, when it comes to weight loss, stress can wreak havoc on your goals.

The good news? Mindful meditation helps you recognize and acknowledge emotions that may be getting in the way of your goals without judgment, guilt, or shame. It may sound simple, but don't undermine its effectiveness! It's been shown to be beneficial for long-term weight loss, helping to promote sustainable healthy lifestyle behaviors and eating habits.

Try this 10-minute Mindful Awareness Meditation with DeAndre Sinette to help you ground down, slow down, and come back to the present.

Day #13: TRADE YOUR COCKTAIL FOR A MOCKTAIL

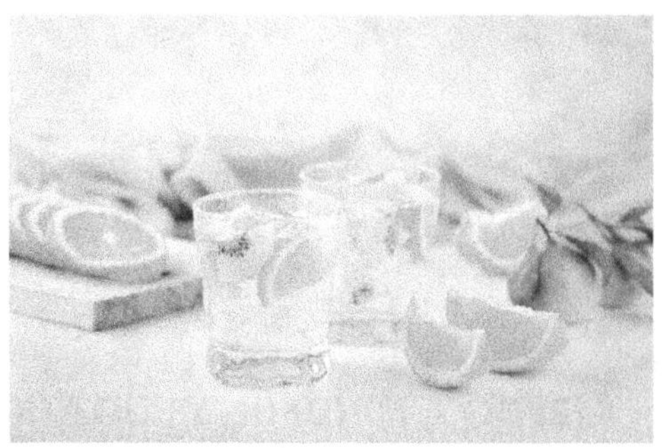

We're not saying you have to give up alcohol forever (unless that's your goal). The occasional drink — when enjoyed in moderation — can be part of a healthy lifestyle, but taking a break from the booze could be a game-changer for your mind, body, and weight loss goals!

Alcohol contains 7 calories per gram, which is a concentrated source of calories — especially considering it's primarily void of additional nutrients. And let's face it — once you start sipping, it can be easy to overindulge.

But fear not — you don't have to miss out! Mocktails make a great substitute for cocktails. Plus, they're incredibly delicious! From Moscow mules to margaritas, there's a healthy mocktail for all your favorite drinks. Did we mention they're easy to whip up at home?

Give this yummy Watermelon Mint Cooler recipe a try, or find some more inspiration here.

Watermelon Mint Cooler
Serves: 1

Ingredients:

Crushed ice
½ cup pure watermelon juice, unsweetened
½ – 1 cup sparkling or seltzer water
1-2 tbsp lime juice, freshly squeezed
Fresh mint, to taste
Directions:

Step #1: Fill the glass with crushed ice.

Step #2: Pour watermelon and lime juice over ice.

Step #3: Top with sparkling water and stir until well mixed.

Step #4: Garnish with fresh lime and mint. Enjoy!

Day #14: AVOID ADDED SUGARS

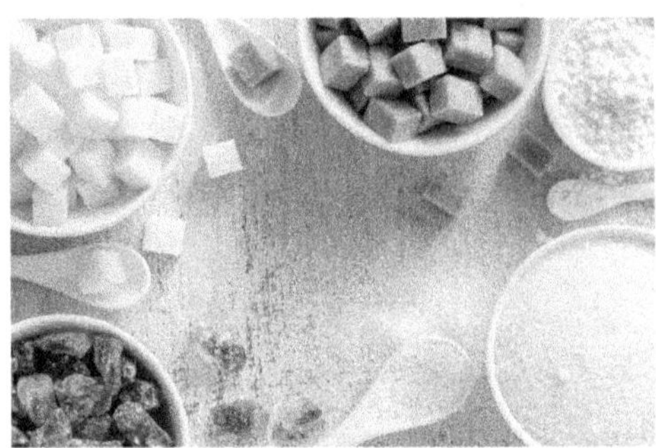

Now that you've got two weeks under your belt, it's time to address a biggie — sugar! Sugar is downright addictive, so if you're struggling to limit your sugar intake, you're certainly not alone.

Start by reading the ingredient label — on everything! From pasta sauce to salad dressing, sugar is hiding in more packaged foods than you think. Start eliminating these foods and instead replace them with healthier swaps. You don't need to avoid sugar in its entirety, but if you're going to consume sugar, stick to whole-food sugar sources.

Options like raw honey, Medjool dates, coconut sugar, and fruit are the least processed, most nutritious sources!

Day #15: PRIORITIZE PROTEIN (AT EVERY MEAL!)

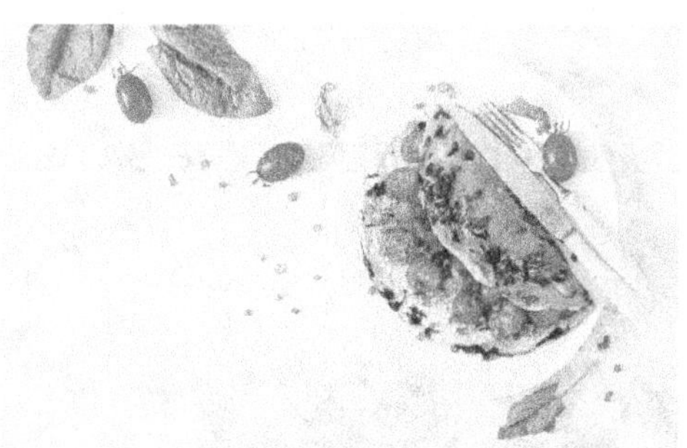

Protein is one of those good-for-you nutrients that's always a good idea — especially if you're trying to lose weight. It helps increase lean muscle mass, boost metabolism, and curb hunger cravings — three very important factors for weight loss! Try to include protein in all your meals today.

Here are some ideas:

Add a tablespoon of nut or seed butter to your smoothie or oatmeal bowl
Top your salad with lean protein, such as grilled salmon, chicken, or tofu
Stir in a spoonful of chia seeds to your overnight oats or baked goods
Add Greek yogurt to sauces, dips, and spreads
Snack on some hard-boiled eggs with a side of veggies or avocado

Day #16: EAT UNTIL YOU'RE SATISFIED

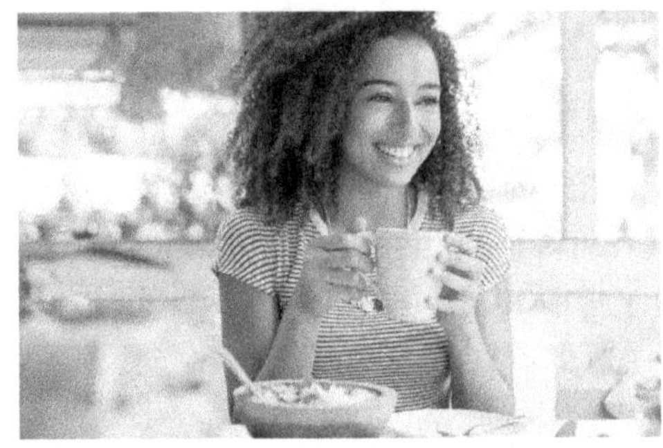

When your meal is full of all the goods, it can be tempting to lick your plate clean and enjoy every last bite! But, you don't HAVE to finish your plate — especially if you're feeling full! Remember: your food isn't going anywhere — you can always save it to enjoy later.

Instead, try to chew your food, eat slowly, and stop when you're 80% full. You should feel satisfied, not stuffed! Try this today and see how you feel.

This weight loss hack is a component of mindful eating, which comes with a long list of benefits (more on this below). Try to listen to your natural hunger cues and tune into how you feel.

Day #17: TRY A NEW HEALTHY RECIPE

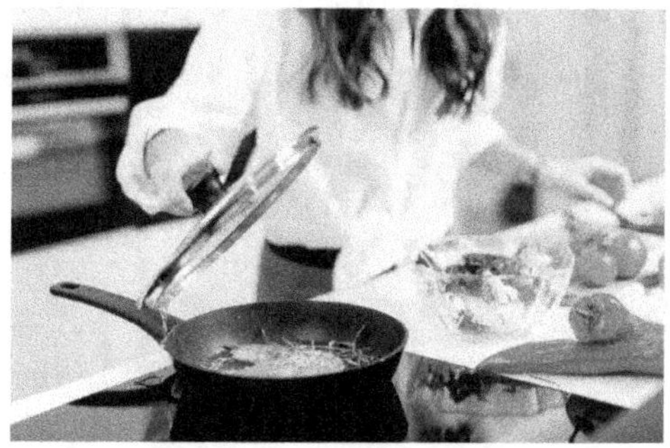

It's easy to get stuck in a cooking rut. Let's face it, eating the same foods is easy and convenient. That said, you'll be more inclined to reach for those tempting snacks if you're bored with your meals. Plus, sticking to the same foods means you're missing out on an abundance of nutrients!

Try something totally new today — it could be completely outside the box, or it could be a recipe you've been dying to try but haven't. Try to do this weekly. It will keep you motivated in the kitchen, you'll load up on a variety of nutrients, and you'll discover new foods. You can even make it a family affair and involve your kids or partner in the process.

Day #18: GIVE YOUR FAVORITE DESSERT A HEALTHY UPGRADE

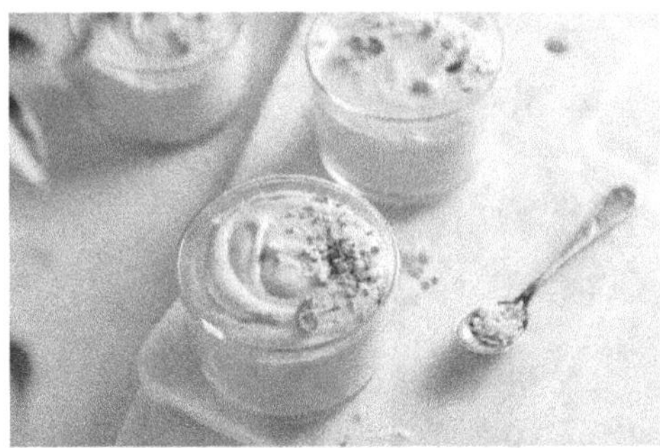

Sweet tooth lovers, listen up! You can still eat dessert and lose weight. In fact, the occasional treat can help prevent binge-eating triggered by excessive dieting and food restriction. That said, you don't need to consume excessive amounts of sugar, fat, and calories to satisfy your sweet tooth cravings. There are so many ways to modify your favorite indulgence and turn it into a guilt-free treat made with good-for-you ingredients.

Treat yourself today! Here are some ideas:

Skip the added sugar and dairy and blend up a naturally-sweetened banana nice cream
Enjoy a 4-ingredient chocolate avocado pudding in place of traditional high-sugar pudding
Whip up a healthy cookie dough froyo made with ingredients like Greek yogurt, almond butter, and cacao nibs
Roll up some no-bake bliss balls and enjoy 1 or 2 as a healthier alternative to cookies.

Day #19: MAKE A NUTRIENT-PACKED SMOOTHIE

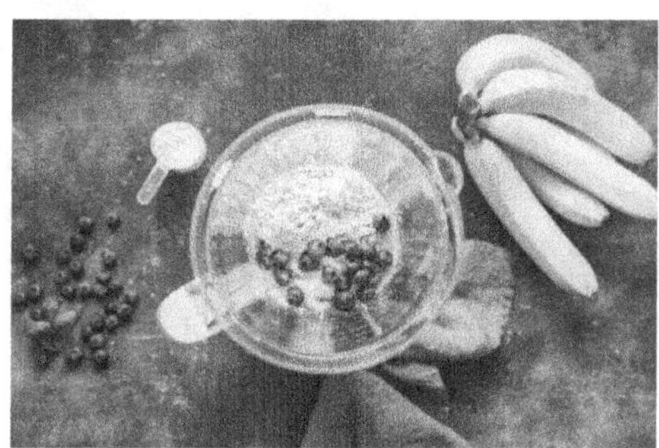

Smoothies are a simple and delicious way to jam-pack a ton of nutrients into one easy-prep meal or snack. Toss in some greens, add a spoonful of superfoods, sneak in some hidden veggies (like cauliflower or zucchini), and blend it up into a weight-loss-friendly meal.

Try this Protein-Packed Banana Berry FitOn Smoothie in place of one of today's meals!

Ingredients:

1 cup frozen berries
½ cup oats
1 tbsp peanut butter
¾ cup Greek yogurt
1½ cups unsweetened almond milk
1 banana, chopped
2 tsp honey
Directions:

Step #1: Add the oats to the blender and pulse a few times until they form a fine flour. Add the remaining ingredients and blend until smooth. Taste test, adjusting any ingredients as needed.

Day #20: EAT THE RAINBOW

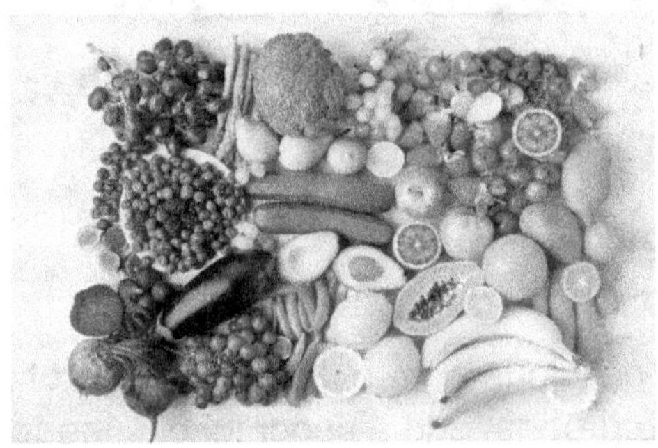

Rather than focus on what to avoid, develop an abundance mindset and consider what foods you can add in! Incorporating an abundance of whole food nutrients rich in various colors is a healthy and sustainable weight loss hack. For today's challenge, try to eat the rainbow. By this, we mean incorporate as many different colored fruits and veggies as you can — the more colors, the more nutrients!

Red-colored fruits & veggies: Rich in lycopene and quercetin to support healthy skin, benefit blood pressure and heart health, blood and support joints.

Yellow & orange-colored fruits & veggies: Rich in lutein and beta carotene to reduce the risk of chronic illness, support eye and skin health, and boost immune health.

Blue & purple-colored fruits & veggies: Rich in anthocyanins, resveratrol, and flavonoids to support brain function, heart health, and healthy aging.

Green-colored fruits & veggies: Rich in chlorophyll, sulforaphane, and antioxidants to detoxify the body, improve immune function, benefit digestion, and fight free radical damage.

Day #21 KEEP A WATER BOTTLE WITH YOU AT ALL TIMES!

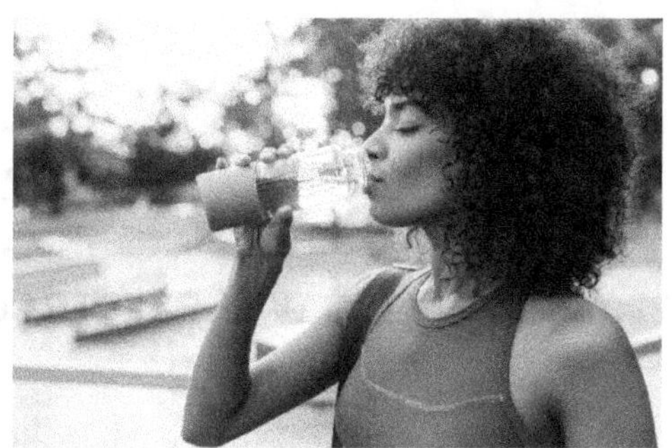

Water is your weight loss BFF. Grab a sustainable water bottle and keep it with you at all times! It will serve as a constant reminder to keep sipping, which can prevent overeating, curb sugar cravings, boost metabolism, and increase satiety.

Day #22: AVOID EATING WHILE DISTRACTED

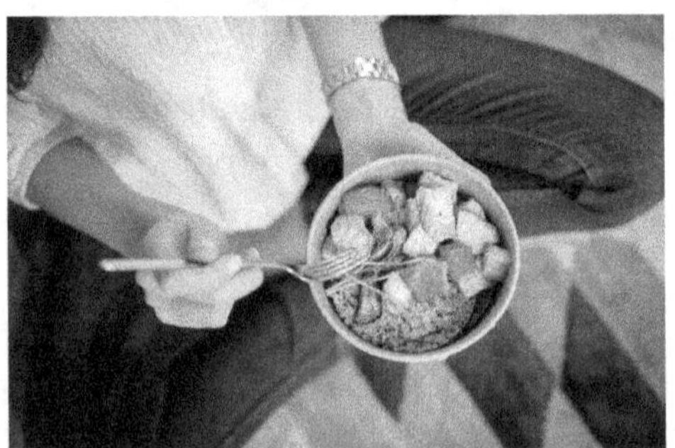

If you're used to eating while walking, driving, watching TV, or working, we challenge you to change your eating habits! Eating while distracted can lead to overeating, both in the moment and later in the day! You'll feel less satiated and satisfied and will be more likely to snack on unhealthy options. So, put the phone away, turn off the TV, close your laptop, and take a seat! Mindful eating is positively associated with weight loss, where it has been shown to reduce the amount of food consumed during meals while also reducing food cravings.

Day #23: BECOME A SMART SNACKER

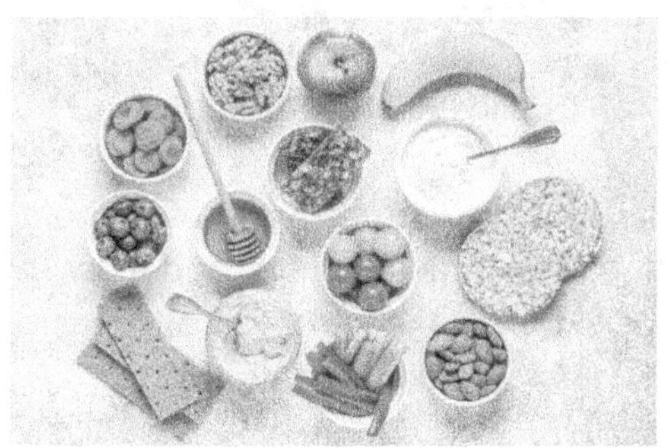

Are snacks standing in the way of you and your weight loss goals? You're not alone! That said, the act of snacking isn't necessarily the problem. Rather, it's the type of snacks you're choosing and the quantity you're consuming! We're looking at you, sugary cereals, late-night ice cream pints, and processed chips.

Challenge yourself to become a smart snacker. Rather than over-consuming calorie-rich foods void of nutrients, choose whole food snacks high in fiber, protein, and healthy fats. And portion them out!

Some ideas:

Homemade energy balls made with nut butter, oats, flax, and chia seeds
Hard-boiled eggs with a side of mashed avocado
Rice cakes with veggies, hummus, and a sprinkle of hemp seeds
A protein-packed snack plate filled with edamame, nuts, and a side of fruit or veggies

Day #24: END THE DAY WITH A WARMING HERBAL TEA

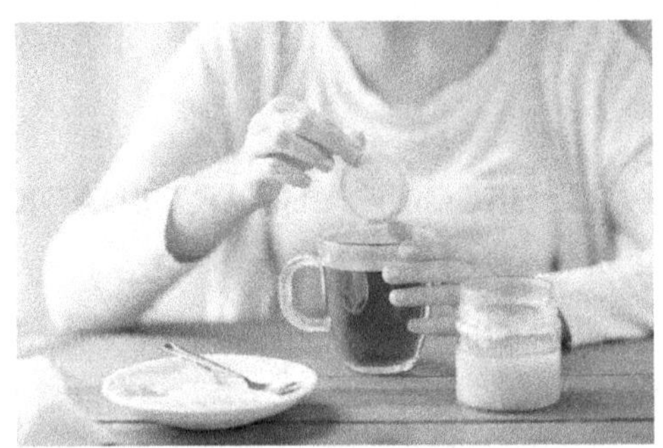

Trade your late-night sweet snack for a warming cup of herbal tea! Certain herbal teas have been shown to benefit digestion, boost metabolism, and aid weight loss. So go ahead, sip all day long! But before you pour a cup, make sure it's caffeine-free (if you're enjoying it as an evening nightcap).

Here are some blends to consider: Oolong, rooibos, ginger, matcha, or dandelion leaf tea.

Day #25: CHECK IN WITH YOUR GOALS & JOURNAL ABOUT HOW YOU FEEL

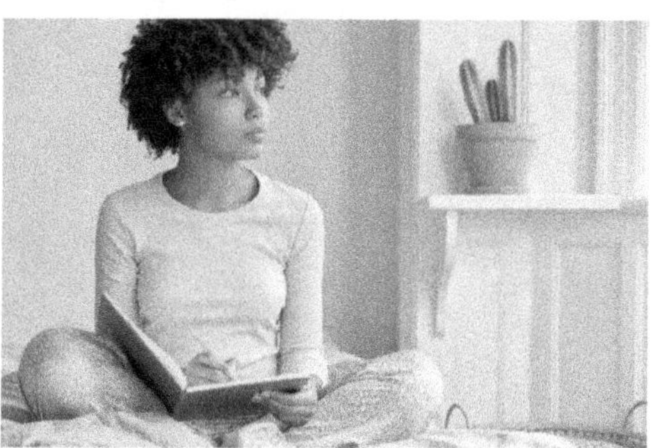

You did it! 25 days of small, actionable habits to help you achieve (and maintain) your weight loss goals. Grab a notebook and pen and reflect on the last month.

Here are some questions and prompts to consider journaling:

How do you feel?
Reflect upon your 'why' — is your motivating weight loss force still the same? Have your goals changed? How do they compare to your Day 1 goals?
What worked really well? What would you do differently?
What was your biggest stressor during this challenge, and how did you work through it?
What healthy habits have made the biggest impact in your day-to-day routine?
List your 5 biggest takeaways
Are there any areas or habits that you want to focus on? Write them down
Write down 3-5 positive affirmations and take time to acknowledge your progress — big or small
Regular self-reflection is one of the most important secrets to long-term weight loss. It helps keep you focused, motivated, and intentional. Plus, it allows you to narrow in on your goals and fine-tune any areas that need improvement or adjustments. By returning to your goals and your 'why,' you're more likely to achieve what you set out to do — both long and short-term!

Keep Going!
You've accomplished so much in these last 25 days, don't stop now! Take these simple weight loss hacks and implement them into your daily routine. You can even give this challenge another go-around and start from scratch! Be proud of all you've accomplished.
Remember: it's a journey!